THE HUMAN BODY IN 3D

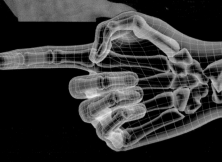

THE LOWER LIMBS IN 3D

rosen publishing's
rosen central

MONICA K. GILL AND
JENNIFER VIEGAS

Published in 2016 by The Rosen Publishing Group, Inc.
29 East 21st Street, New York, NY 10010

First Edition

Library of Congress Cataloging-in-Publication Data

Gill, Monica K.
The lower limbs in 3D/Monica K. Gill and Jennifer Viegas.
    pages cm.—(The human body in 3D)
Includes bibliographical references and index.
ISBN 978-1-4994-3601-3 (library bound)—ISBN 978-1-4994-3602-0 (pbk.)—
ISBN 978-1-4994-3604-4 (6-pack)
1. Leg—Juvenile literature. I. Viegas, Jennifer. II. Title.
QM549.G55 2016
611'.98—dc23

2015000141

Manufactured in the United States of America

CONTENTS

INTRODUCTION 4

CHAPTER ONE
THE PELVIC GIRDLE AND UPPER LEG 7

CHAPTER TWO
THE KNEE: THE BODY'S LARGEST JOINT....................... 18

CHAPTER THREE
THE LOWER LEG 28

CHAPTER FOUR
THE ANKLE AND FOOT 41

GLOSSARY 53

FOR MORE INFORMATION 56

FOR FURTHER READING 59

INDEX 61

INTRODUCTION

Consider for a moment how much you move from day to day. You walk around your home and from your room to your front door or garage. You might run from class to class, and perhaps you play a sport after school. Wherever you go, chances are, you will need to use your lower limbs. These limbs make up, as the name suggests, the lower half of the body. They give the body balance and mobility. Without them, you could not walk, run, jump, dance, or kick a ball. You might have to inch along like a worm or slither like a snake.

The lower limbs consist of the pelvic girdle, which is formed by the hip bones, your thighs, your lower legs, and your feet. The bones and muscles of the lower limbs support the body's weight as it moves. In conjunction with other parts of the body, lower limb muscles contract, extend, flex, absorb impact, and more. Together they give the body the ability to move in many different ways, over different terrains, and across short and long distances.

If you compare the human body to the bodies of many other animals, you might appreciate just how much your own lower limbs are capable of. Humans have just two legs to support themselves. Cats and dogs distribute their weight through

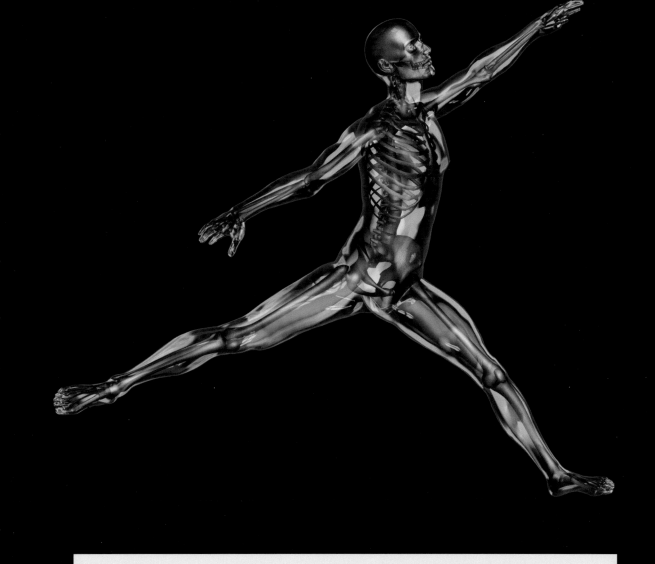

The human body is capable of a wide range of motion, thanks in large part to the lower limbs.

four legs, while insects might have six or eight legs that carry them. They are therefore more stable and can balance better than bipedal, or two-legged, animals. Most four-legged animals can also move much faster than humans; cheetahs, for example, can run 75 miles (120 kilometers) per hour. But the lower limbs of the human body give us some major advantages. The body exerts less energy when walking upright on two legs instead of down on four or more. And despite being less stable and moving more slowly, humans are capable of a wide range of activities, including climbing and swimming. Few other animals can sustain two-legged movement the way humans can.

Lower limb movement is carefully orchestrated by many different bones, muscles, joints, nerves, tendons, ligaments, and other body parts. The human foot alone has twenty-six bones, thirty-three joints, and over one hundred muscles. There are some major bones and muscles to keep in mind, however. Among others, important bones in the leg include the femur (thighbone) and the tibia (shinbone). Metatarsals are major bones in the toes. Major muscles in the leg include the gluteus muscles, the quadriceps, and the hamstring muscles.

Lower limbs are remarkably resilient—from infanthood to adulthood, lower limbs grow and change to support all of our various activities. Like other parts of the body, these limbs are susceptible to injury, disease, and other damage. But with a proper balance of nutrition, care, and exercise, you can help make sure that they remain healthy, strong, and flexible for years to come.

CHAPTER ONE

THE PELVIC GIRDLE AND UPPER LEG

The lower limbs are made up of six primary sections: the pelvic girdle, the upper leg, the knee, the lower leg, the ankle, and the foot. Each part functions differently from the others, but all work together to give the body mobility and balance. The pelvic girdle, which is part of the hip, and the upper leg make up the top portion of the lower limbs. The muscles in these areas help the body move side to side and back and forth.

THE HIP AND PELVIC GIRDLE

The hip bone, also called the pelvis, holds the hip and legs in place and cradles the bladder, the sac that holds liquid waste from the body. The bones that look like giant mouse ears at the top form the ilium, or the pelvic girdle. The pelvic girdle is what can be felt

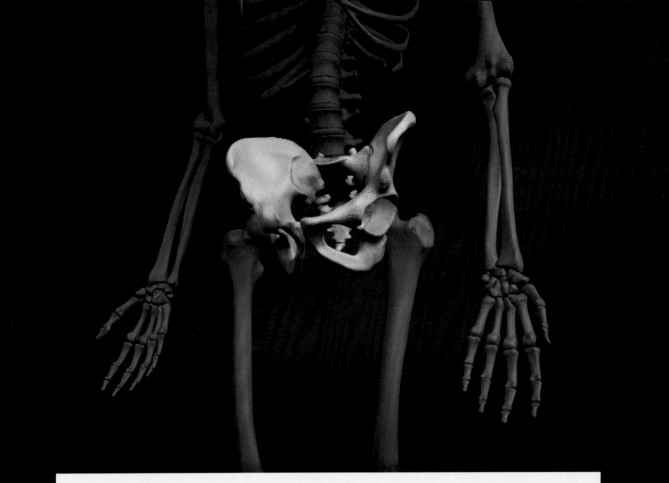

The pelvic girdle is made up of two hip bones, each of which consists of three bones: the ilium, the ischium, and the pubis.

when the hands are placed on the hips. The upside down triangle in the middle that you would feel with your thumbs consists of the sacrum and coccyx, or tailbone. These are several vertebrae that are fused together. Vertebrae, in turn, are small rings of bone that protect the spine and form the backbone. Bend the back slightly and feel the vertebrae along the spine.

The legs are attached to the hip in a socket called the acetabulum. The acetabula (plural for acetabulum) lie at opposite ends of the hip bone and face outward. This arrangement improves balance and range of movement. Imagine if the acetabula were stuck together at the front of the hip. People would be forced to take tiny tiptoe steps, leaning backward for balance! The acetabulum has an inward curve that accommodates the ball-shaped end of the femur, or thighbone. Together, the round head of the femur and the acetabulum create what is known as a ball-and-socket joint.

SYNOVIAL JOINTS

Joints are places where two bones meet. The body has many joints. For example, take a look at your fingers. Each finger has three joints. One is near where the knuckle meets the hand and the other two joints are where the finger bends. Feel how these joints define separate bones in a finger.

There are three main types of joints in the body: moveable ones, called synovial joints; fixed ones, called fibrous joints; and cartilaginous joints, places where bone meets with cartilage, a flexible, gristlelike material. "Synovial" refers to a membrane, or thin sheet of tissue, that lines certain joints. This tissue releases synovial fluid, which is a slippery substance that makes moving easier. Synovial fluid is similar to the oil used to repair a squeaky door with a tight hinge.

Synovial joints can be further divided into different types, depending on how the joints move and work. The ball-and-socket joint in the pelvis is one such type. It allows for a full range of movement. Thanks to this kind of joint in the pelvis, people can swing their legs around in a circle. Keep this in mind when watching people

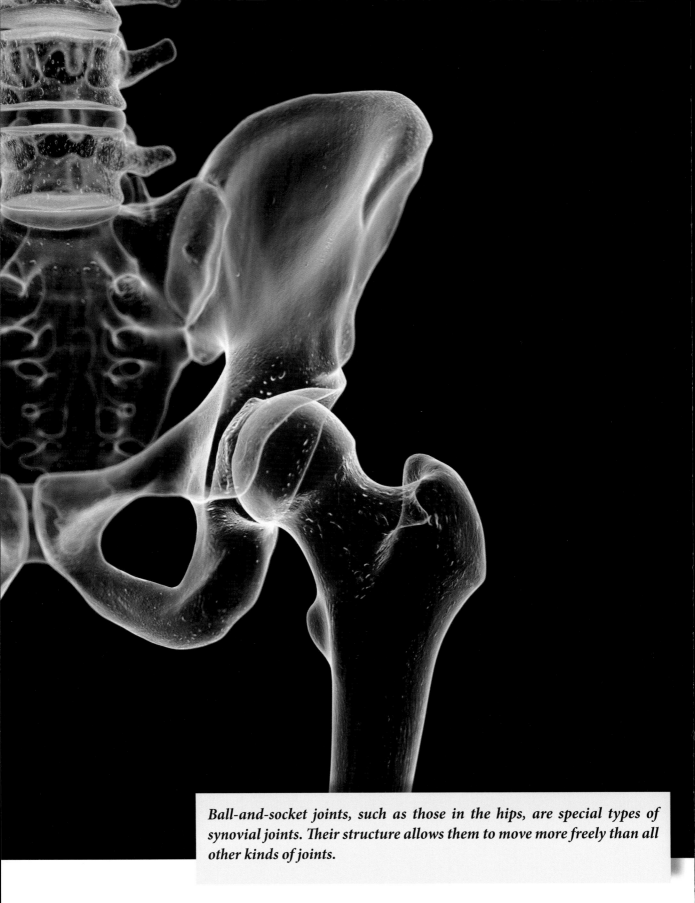

Ball-and-socket joints, such as those in the hips, are special types of synovial joints. Their structure allows them to move more freely than all other kinds of joints.

twist and turn their legs while playing sports, such as football and basketball, or while dancing and skating. With every move of the upper leg, the circular top of the femur bone rotates in the ball-and-socket joint. The synovial fluid ensures that such movements are smooth and without friction, or rubbing, which can cause damage.

THE ROLE OF NERVES

Nerves are bundles of special tissue that carry messages to and from the brain. The spinal cord at the center of the back, which is protected by the vertebrae, serves as a collection center for nerves within the body. All nerves originate at the spinal cord and branch out to every part of the body, from the tips of the fingers to the bottom of the feet. Around the hip area, nerves look like large sprigs of grass sprouting from the spine.

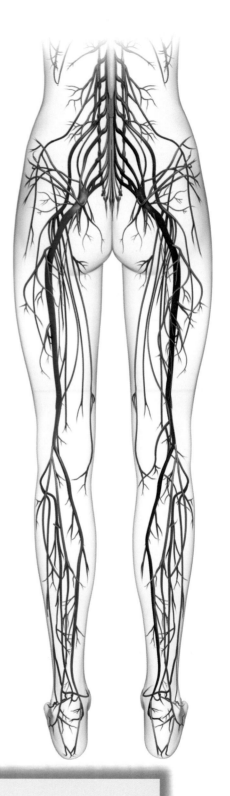

The sciatic nerve, highlighted in purple, is the body's largest and thickest nerve. It descends from the lower spine through the back of the leg, branching into the tibial nerve just above the knee.

Through electrical impulses that release chemicals called neurotransmitters, nerves can control movement. In a chain reaction, individual nerve cells, called neurons, pass electrical impulses to each other until the contained message reaches its destination. For example, lift a leg now. In that split second, the brain sends a message down through the spinal cord and to the leg, with countless neuron exchanges occurring along the way. At the leg, the neurons instruct muscles there to move.

THE UPPER LEG

The area between the hip and knee—the upper leg—is the thigh. Most animals with legs, including humans, have thighs. In fact, ham and leg of lamb are cuts of meat that come from the thighs of pigs and lambs. Thighs are thick, fleshy, and muscular. Thigh muscles are needed to support and move the body.

UPPER LEG MUSCLES

Muscles are strong and powerful tissues that are responsible for all body movements. When stimulated by nerves, muscles contract, or shorten and become tighter, which pulls bones closer together. An important point to remember is that muscles can pull, but they cannot push. This means that different muscles are required for varying movements.

Tensor fasciae latae

Gracilis

Sartorius

Rectus femoris

Vastus lateralis

Vastus medialis

Four different muscles in the thigh make up the large muscle group called the quadriceps. These are the rectus femoris, the vastus lateralis, the vastus medialis, and the vastus intermedius.

The gluteus meteus muscle at each pelvic ball-and-socket joint controls the turning, rotating, and extending of the thigh. Just behind the gluteus meteus is the gluteus maximus. This big muscle aids the gluteus meteus in extending and rotating the thigh. It also braces the knee. The sartorius muscle, which wraps around the front of the thigh, is the longest muscle in the body. It flexes and rotates the thigh and leg. Two of the main muscles at the front of the thigh are the rectus femoris and the vastus lateralis.

Anterior view of leg muscles

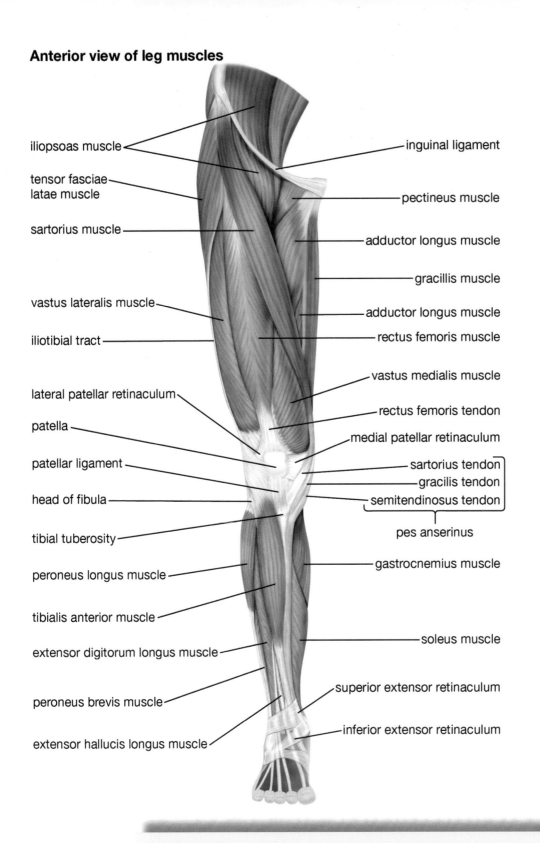

iliopsoas muscle

tensor fasciae latae muscle

sartorius muscle

vastus lateralis muscle

iliotibial tract

lateral patellar retinaculum

patella

patellar ligament

head of fibula

tibial tuberosity

peroneus longus muscle

tibialis anterior muscle

extensor digitorum longus muscle

peroneus brevis muscle

extensor hallucis longus muscle

inguinal ligament

pectineus muscle

adductor longus muscle

gracillis muscle

adductor longus muscle

rectus femoris muscle

vastus medialis muscle

rectus femoris tendon

medial patellar retinaculum

sartorius tendon
gracilis tendon
semitendinosus tendon

pes anserinus

gastrocnemius muscle

soleus muscle

superior extensor retinaculum

inferior extensor retinaculum

Leg muscles can be large, such as those in the thigh, or small, such as those in the feet. Many muscles work together in groups to perform a range of functions, including moving or balancing the body.

HOW STRONG IS YOUR THIGH?

All healthy individuals have strong thigh muscles that carry the weight of the body and move the legs. Here is a fun way to measure thigh muscle strength. With permission, take a bathroom scale, preferably one that is no longer needed to measure weight, and place it between the knees. Now, squeeze as hard as possible. Have someone write down the scale reading. The number is a measurement of how strong the inner thigh muscles are. Exercise can strengthen muscles, so try to increase the number over time by exercising the thigh and leg muscles regularly.

Like big computer cables, muscles are made out of thick bands that contain smaller fibers. Within each muscle fiber—about the size of a strand of hair—are even smaller myofibrils. These, in turn, contain ultra tiny threads, called myosin and actin filaments, that interact and allow for muscle contraction and relaxation. While the process is complex, basically the filaments move closer together during contraction, causing the muscle to pull. During relaxation, the filaments move farther apart, and the muscle relaxes.

CONNECTING MUSCLE TO BONE

Underneath the skin of the thigh, the thigh muscles can be seen as thick, fleshy strands. If the leg were lifted, these strands would contract, causing the leg to move in a certain direction depending

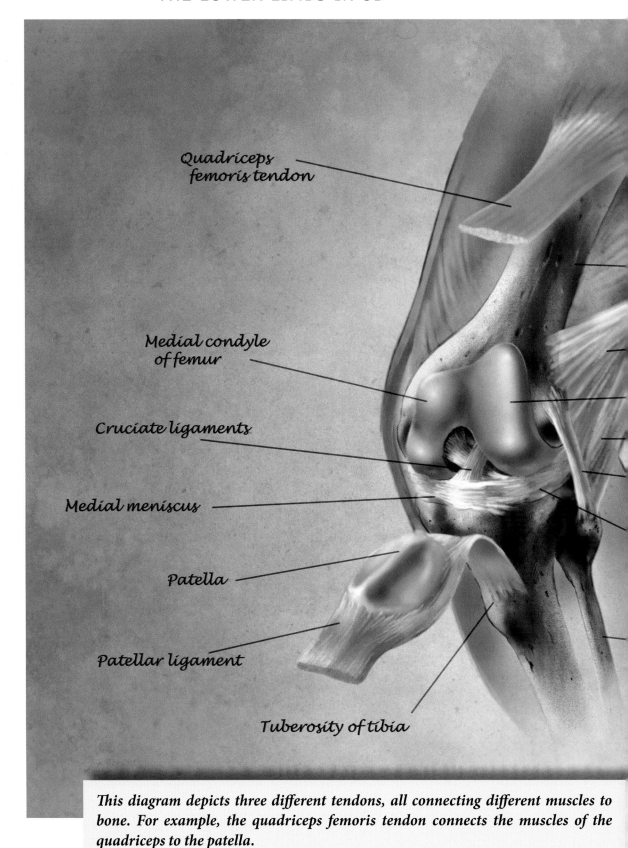

Quadriceps
femoris tendon

Medial condyle
of femur

Cruciate ligaments

Medial meniscus

Patella

Patellar ligament

Tuberosity of tibia

This diagram depicts three different tendons, all connecting different muscles to bone. For example, the quadriceps femoris tendon connects the muscles of the quadriceps to the patella.

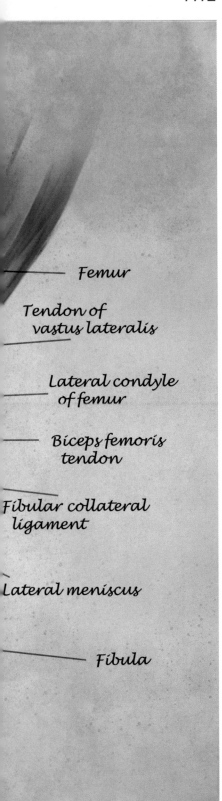

Femur

Tendon of
vastus lateralis

Lateral condyle
of femur

Biceps femoris
tendon

Fibular collateral
ligament

Lateral meniscus

Fibula

on what muscle was used. You would also see white bands attached to the ends of the thigh muscles. These are tendons.

Tendons connect muscles to bones. Whenever a muscle contracts, the tendon pulls on a bone, which allows for movement. While the muscle areas of the thigh contain several nerve endings and are supplied with a lot of blood, the tendons are, for the most part, inactive. They are like very strong puppet strings. To control a puppet, someone must tug, or stretch and shorten, the string, causing the attached puppet to move. In the case of tendons, muscles stretch and shorten. The attached tendons then respond to this activity by moving. Bones at the end are like puppets. They have no motion by themselves but simply react to muscle contractions transmitted through tendons.

Tendons, also sometimes called sinews, are made up of very strong connective tissue. Although tendons are located in the body and not on its surface, it is possible to feel what a tendon is like. Place a hand at the back of a knee and swing the lower leg back and forth. The stretching and relaxing sensation is actually the hamstring tendon, connected to the hamstring muscles of the thigh, moving the lower leg bones back and forth.

CHAPTER TWO

THE KNEE: THE BODY'S LARGEST JOINT

The femur is the only bone in the upper leg. It is the body's largest bone, and it connects to the body's largest joint, the knee. The knee connects the femur to the tibia, the major bone of the lower leg. The knee is made up of many different parts—bones, ligaments, and cartilage—which help it endure the stresses that result from supporting the body's weight.

KNEE FUNCTION

To understand the amount of work the knee does, think about a door joint for a minute. Imagine what would happen to the door if it were slammed open and shut all day. At the very least, the joint would require constant maintenance. Over time it would probably have to be repaired or replaced.

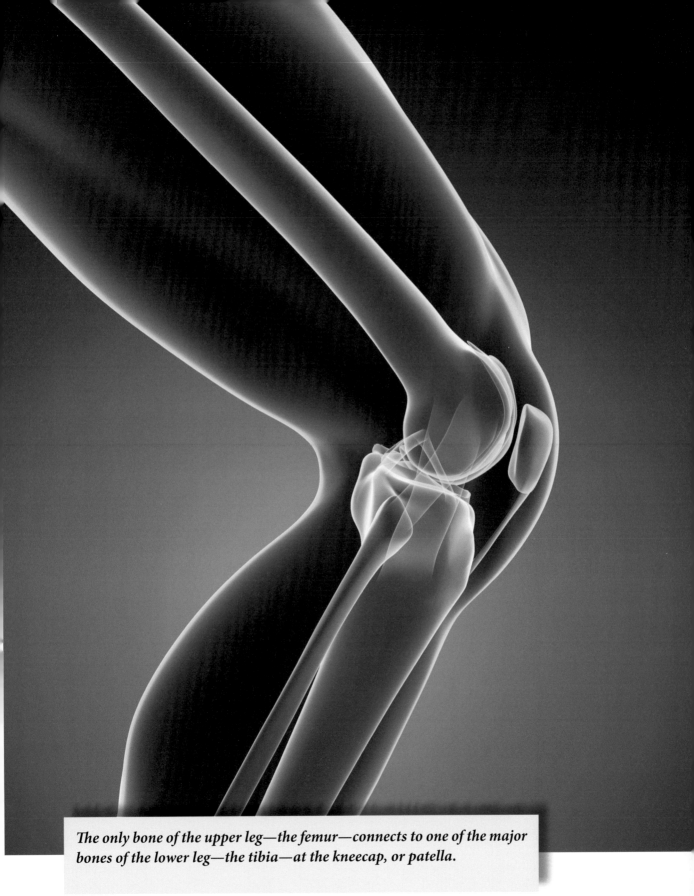

The only bone of the upper leg—the femur—connects to one of the major bones of the lower leg—the tibia—at the kneecap, or patella.

Knees take this kind of abuse every day. Think of how many times the knees must bend. They bend when a person sits, walks, kicks, runs, and even sleeps. Because of all of the potential wear and tear, knees have a more complex construction than other joints.

In the same way that the hip bone has grooves where it meets the thighbone, the top of the tibia is slightly concave, or cup shaped, where it meets the femur. Given all of the movement in this region, these two bones could grind against each other without protection. Cartilage takes care of this by forming a protective surface at the knee where the leg bones meet.

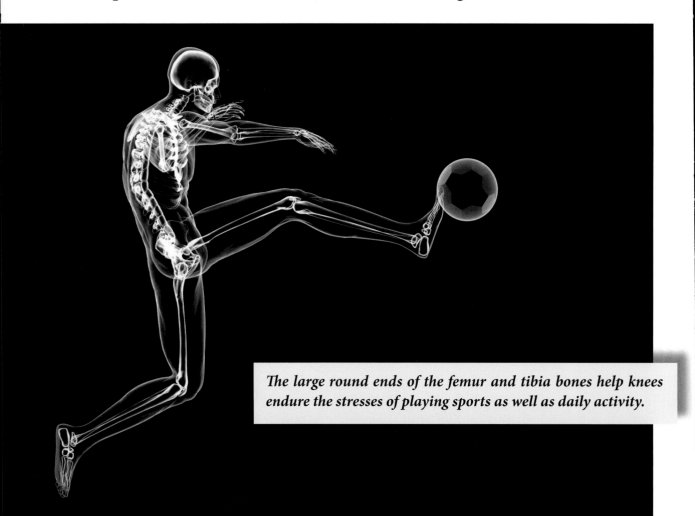

The large round ends of the femur and tibia bones help knees endure the stresses of playing sports as well as daily activity.

THE ROLE OF CARTILAGE

Cartilage is a tough, yet flexible, part of the body that is mostly found in joints, such as the knee, and other places where flexibility is essential. Most of the nose and ears are cartilage, which is why these areas respond easily to touch and motion, such as when the nostrils are pinched together or when the ears move when a sweater or shirt is pulled over them.

Cartilage is constructed like a net with cells and fibers running through it. These fibers are made from proteins called collagen and elastin. Manufacturers of cosmetics often refer to these terms because the protein fibers, also found in skin, can degrade with age and are associated with wrinkle formation. Collagen is also what mostly makes the dark meat in chicken different than the white meat. Just as humans have a lot of collagen in the leg cartilage, birds also have it in their wings and legs.

In images of the knee, cartilage can be seen between the thigh and calf bones. The top disk of cartilage is called the medial meniscus, while the one that rests over the tibia is called the lateral meniscus. Together they are called menisci. The knee can function without the protection of cartilage, but not always as smoothly. Athletes often suffer torn cartilage, and the cartilage has to be removed. Sometimes this can lead to arthritis and other problems later in life.

Synovial fluid surrounds the cartilage and joint area of the knee. The word "synovial" comes from the Greek word for "egg white," which this fluid somewhat resembles. In addition to the

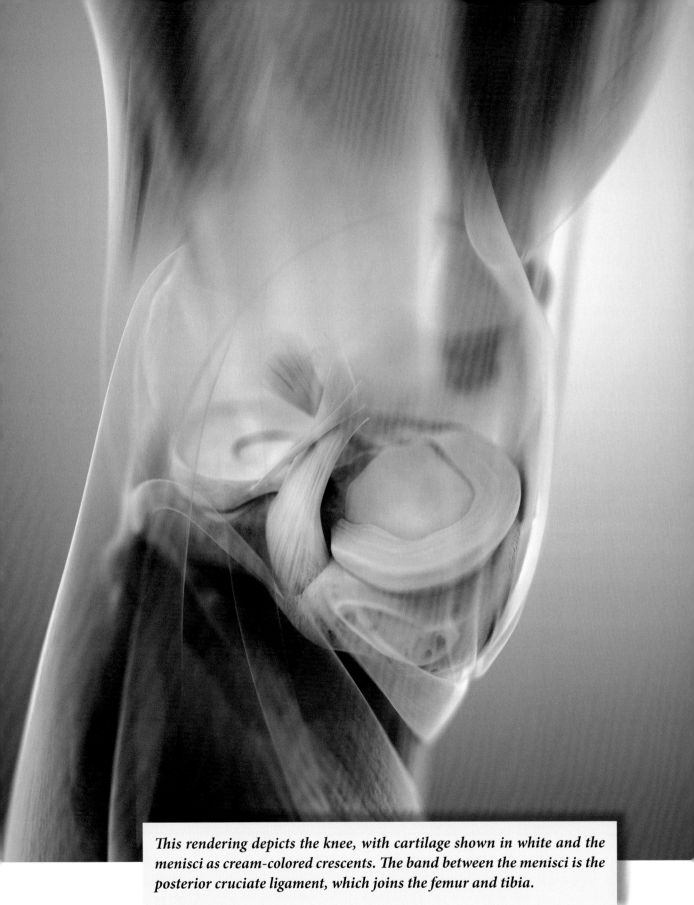

This rendering depicts the knee, with cartilage shown in white and the menisci as cream-colored crescents. The band between the menisci is the posterior cruciate ligament, which joins the femur and tibia.

UNDERSTANDING THE KNEE-JERK REACTION

Reflexes are automatic reactions that the body performs to protect itself. One of the most well known is called the knee-jerk reflex. Doctors often test this reflex to see how well a patient's muscles and nerves are working. They do this by tapping the tendon below the kneecap. Nerves in the tendon travel to the spinal cord, which sends a signal to the muscles at the front of the thigh to contract, causing the knee to jerk forward. The patient becomes aware of the response later, after a message has had time to travel to the brain.

oil-like synovial lubricant, two other sacs of fluid, called bursae, rest between the femur and tibia. The bursae are like little cushions that relieve stress and strain on the joint. Ligaments are in the middle of the joint, too, and also lie on either side of the knee.

CONNECTING BONE TO BONE

Ligaments are similar to tendons, except that they link bones to other bones and are made of more flexible tissue. Without ligaments, bones in the body would easily become dislocated, like a model airplane that was not glued together properly. While ligaments hold bones together, they also allow for movement. Try walking without bending the knees. It is awkward and not easy.

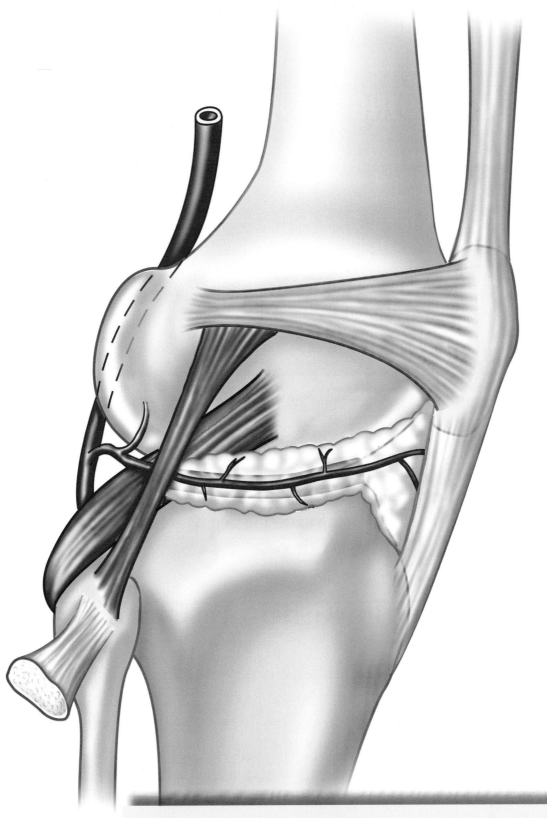

An intricate system of ligaments can be found in the knee. This rendering depicts four ligaments: the patellar ligament (white), the medial patellofemoral ligament (green), the lateral collateral ligament (blue), and the posterior cruciate ligament (purple).

The ligaments in the knee hold the bones of the leg together but still allow the knee joint to bend. The posterior cruciate ligament and anterior cruciate ligament hold the knee together at the joint, while the tibia collateral ligament at the front of the knee and the fibular collateral ligament at the back keep the legs straight and help to prevent the knee from bending backward.

The kneecap is like a built-in kneepad. It is actually a disk-shaped bone, called the patella. Tendons in the body do not usually have bones, but the patella is an exception, as it is part of the tendon of the quadriceps muscle in the thigh. The patella protects this tendon from wearing down due to the joint bending.

The joint at the knee is called a hinge joint. Unlike the ball-and-socket joint at the hips, which allows for a full range of movement, the knee can

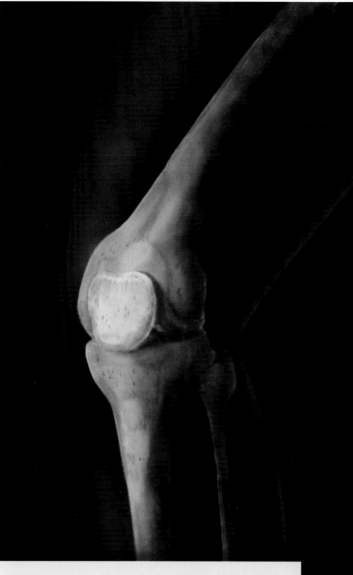

The kneecap, or patella, is a bone found at the end of the femur that helps keep the tibia in place when the leg bends.

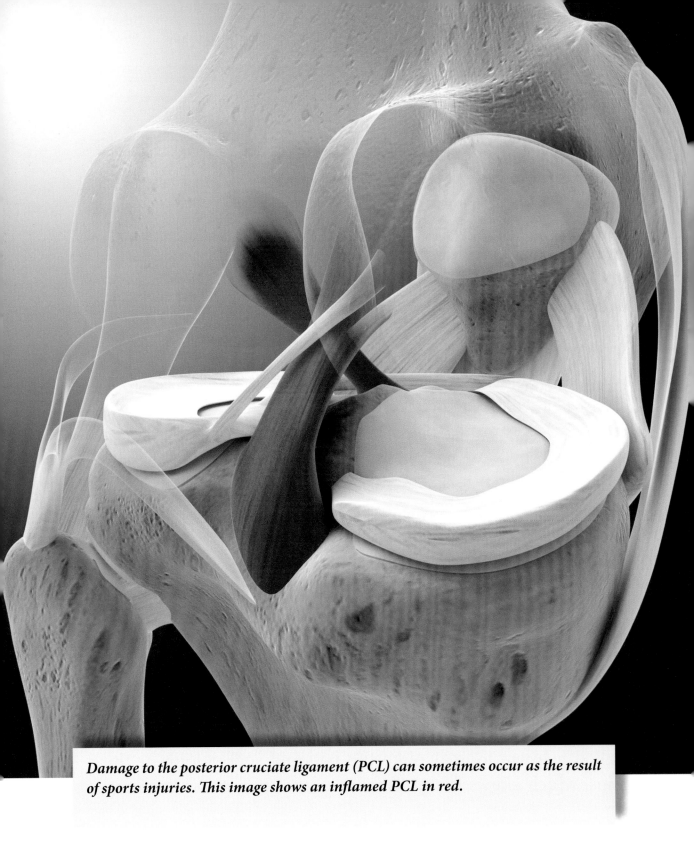

Damage to the posterior cruciate ligament (PCL) can sometimes occur as the result of sports injuries. This image shows an inflamed PCL in red.

only move back and forth. The knee bends in the same way as the pages of a book open and close. The knee does not have to swing around in a circle, as the entire leg can move the knee along with it. Also, the hinge mechanism allows the knees to lock in place so that a person may stand with little effort. Standing up straight with both feet on the ground is not only best for the spine, but it also puts less strain on the knees.

As the largest and heaviest joint, the knee is also the body's most vulnerable one. Although well protected by cartilage, synovial fluid, the bursae, and ligaments, the knee should still be guarded during periods of active use, such as when playing football or volleyball, with kneepads or some other form of protection. Think of all of the great sports stars that have had to curtail their careers because of knee problems. The knee is injured more than any other joint, but proper care can help to prevent it from sustaining damage.

CHAPTER THREE

THE LOWER LEG

The lower leg is found below the knee. The lower leg bones are the tibia (shinbone) and fibula, which is next to the tibia. The tibia and fibula form the front part of the leg. The back portion of the lower leg is called the calf. The calf muscles are connected to the heel by the Achilles tendon. The muscles of the lower leg do many things, including helping us walk and helping the leg move up and down. They even control certain movements of the feet, which are found below the lower leg.

BONE DEVELOPMENT

The three major bones of the leg—the femur, tibia, and fibula—along with the other 203 bones in the body, have a unique structure that makes them, pound for pound, more sturdy and strong than concrete, wood, and even steel. Steel girders hold up giant buildings, including skyscrapers, so imagine how strong human bones—which must support the whole body—are. While the inner structure of bones can slightly vary, depending on where

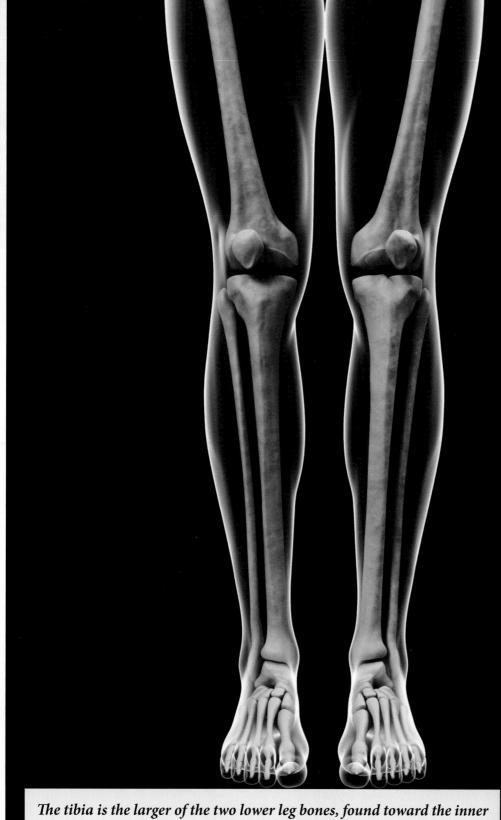

The tibia is the larger of the two lower leg bones, found toward the inner part of the leg. A membrane connects the tibia to the outer lower leg bone, the fibula.

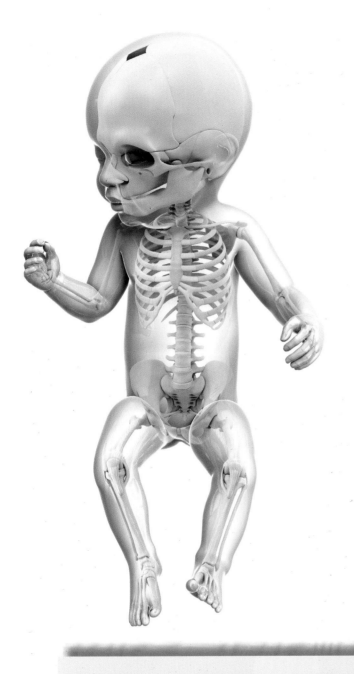

Human babies are born with curved legs, which reflects the position they assumed in the womb. They gain strength in their leg bones after they begin walking, which helps the legs straighten.

the bones are located, the basic components remain the same.

Before birth, the bones of a baby in the womb are made of flexible cartilage. At birth, the cartilage has developed into hard bone. While bones are strong, they are light and not solid. The exterior is often referred to as hard bone. It is actually a tough substance made up of numerous cells. The cells, or the building blocks of all living things, link together to form rings around small holes that can be detected under a microscope. The holes allow blood to pass through and nourish the bone.

Blood cells are created in the honeycomblike centers of many bones. There marrow, a material similar to jelly, falls into two different types: red

MYSTERIOUS RAYS

Our ability to understand the structure of the human body, and to diagnose and cure the illnesses of living patients, really began with the German physicist William Konrad Roentgen (1845–1923) and the mysterious rays he discovered in his laboratory on the winter evening of November 5, 1895.

Roentgen became very interested in the new phenomenon of cathode rays. Earlier scientists had noticed that when an electric current flowed across an open gap inside a glass tube from which the air had been removed, the tube began to fluoresce, or glow. Roentgen repeated this experiment, but he went a step further. He covered the glass tube with a layer of black cardboard so that no light could escape. When he turned on the current, he was amazed to discover that a sample of a barium compound on another table some distance from the cathode ray tube had begun to glow, even though no light had escaped from the glass tube. Some invisible ray, more powerful than light, had penetrated the black cardboard, traveled across the laboratory, and stimulated the fluorescent properties of the barium compound.

Roentgen named these strange rays X-rays because in science, "X" stands for the unknown, and Roentgen had no idea what these rays were. Soon Roentgen was exposing all sorts of materials to these rays and exploring their ability to penetrate some solid objects. Using photographic film, he produced a picture of the bones in his wife's hand.

Soon after, X-rays were all the rage. Only four days after their discovery, American doctors used X-rays to locate a bullet in a patient's leg. The earliest uses of X-rays were in the diagnosis of tuberculosis and cancer. Unfortunately, it took several decades for people to realize that X-rays could damage human tissue. Many doctors and researchers developed radiation burns and cancerous

(continued on the next page)

(continued from the previous page)

tumors, and more than one hundred people died before the danger was recognized. In 1901, Roentgen received the prestigious Nobel Prize for his discovery.

Today X-rays are still an essential tool for doctors, but we also have much more sophisticated techniques for seeing inside the human body without surgery. We have computerized axial tomography (CAT), positron emission tomography (PET), and magnetic resonance imaging (MRI). These techniques create three-dimensional images of internal organs by digitally assembling the data from hundreds of individual scans and show degrees of detail impossible with X-rays. Nevertheless, it all began with an unexpected flicker of light in a dark laboratory.

and yellow. Red marrow makes red blood cells, which help to distribute oxygen throughout the body. Red marrow also produces germ-fighting white blood cells and platelets, which help blood to clot. Yellow marrow, on the other hand, stores fat and distributes it around the body as needed.

Bones keep growing until about the time a person reaches the age of twenty. That is one reason why people continue to get taller through their teens. Bones also rejuvenate themselves, up until the age of thirty-five or so, creating new bone to replace older, damaged spots. After thirty-five, however, this repair process slows down.

Bones store minerals, such as calcium. Like fat from yellow marrow, bones release the minerals when they are needed by

The tibia carries most of the body's weight, but because the tibia and fibula are connected, a fracture in one usually indicates a fracture of the other.

other parts of the body. As a person ages, a lot of the minerals and collagen have already left the bone, which is why older people sometimes suffer from brittle bones and are vulnerable to bone fractures. It is often necessary for such individuals to take calcium supplements, to help deter this aging process.

Despite the fact that they can be broken, bones can often miraculously heal themselves. The healing process begins almost

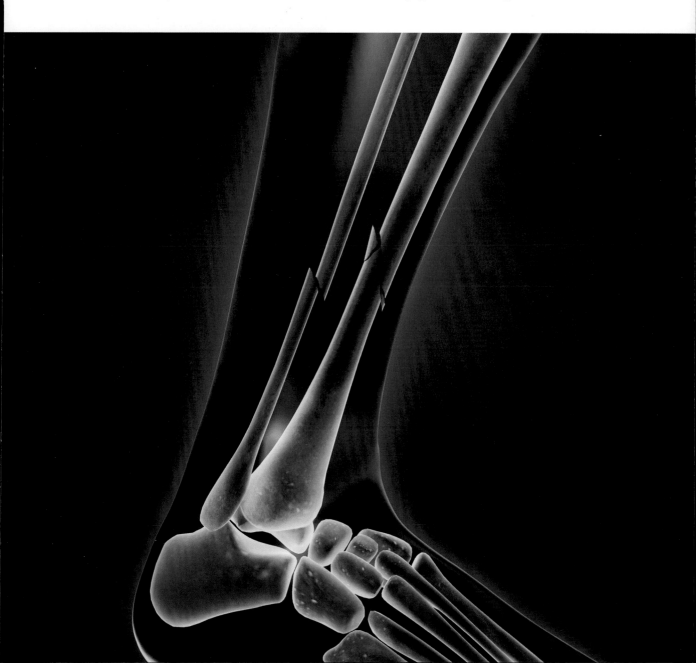

immediately. About an hour after a break, blood oozes out of the broken ends to form a clot. Approximately two days later, bone cells called fibroblasts and osteoblasts string together, forming a loose connection between the broken ends. Gradually, other cells fill in the open spaces and the bone hardens. After about three months, most broken bones have fully mended. To help this happen, doctors often put a cast over the affected area, which holds the bones in place and makes sure the broken parts join together properly.

LOWER LEG MUSCLES

The thigh muscles are connected to bones in the lower leg. Major muscles of the shin area at the front of the lower leg include the peroneus longus muscle, which

Peroneus longus

Tibialis anterior

Extensor digitorum longu

Extensor hallucis longus

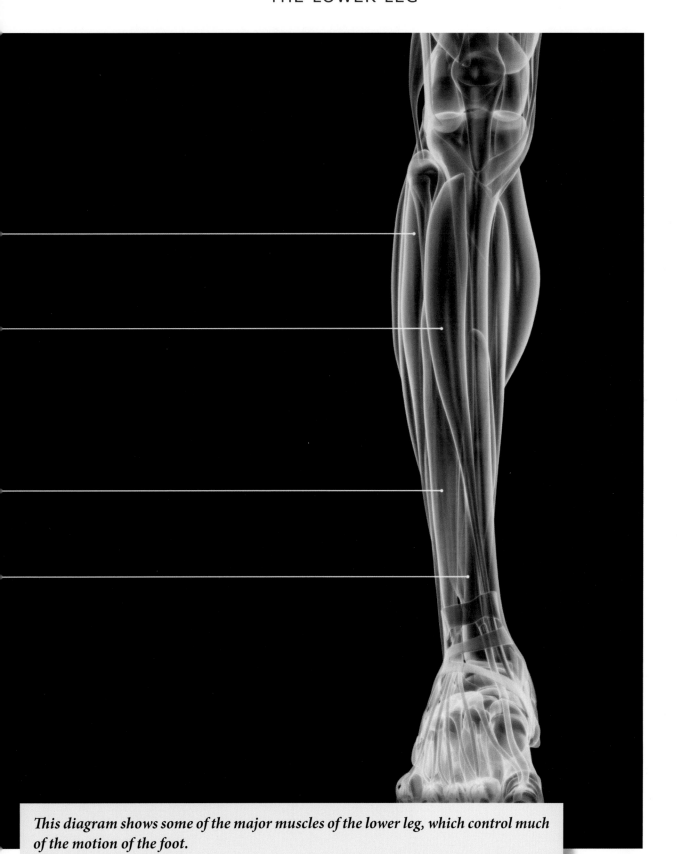

This diagram shows some of the major muscles of the lower leg, which control much of the motion of the foot.

EXERCISE AND LEG MUSCLES

Weight lifters and bodybuilders often have huge leg muscles that bulge and ripple underneath the skin. Interestingly enough, these individuals have the same number of muscle fibers as a couch potato who rarely exercises. Well-trained athletes, however, have larger muscle fibers that contain more actin and myosin. They also develop more connective tissue and have stronger bones and tendons, which is why they can lift heavy objects. While weight lifting may not be for everyone, regular exercise is important for maintaining the health of muscles, keeping body fat to a minimum, and ensuring strong legs for years to come.

aids in walking; the tibialis anterior muscle, which moves the foot up; and the soleus muscle, which flexes the foot down. A major muscle of the calf area at the back of the lower leg is the gastrocnemius muscle. Like the soleus muscle, it helps to flex the foot into a downward position. It also can flex the entire leg.

THE ACHILLES TENDON

A side view of the lower leg reveals the Achilles tendon, also sometimes called the Achilles heel. It looks like a slender white triangle that runs from the back of the leg to the back of the foot. As with all tendons, the job of the Achilles tendon is to link muscle to bone. The Achilles tendon links the large gastrocnemius muscle in the calf of the leg to bone in the foot.

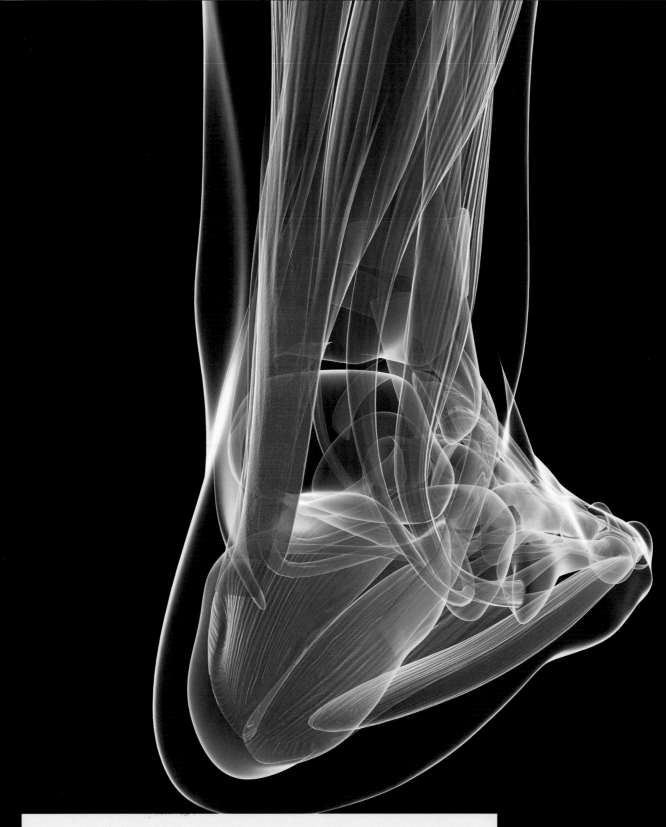

When the muscles of the calf contract, the Achilles tendon, highlighted here in red, helps lift the foot, allowing us to perform a range of motion, including walking and running.

The Achilles tendon is the strongest tendon in the entire body. Because it is so big and strong, this tendon can be easily felt. Try to feel it now, by placing a hand at the calf where the leg meets the foot. Now, point the toes of that foot and bend the foot into an upward position. The tightening sensation is the tendon pulling on the foot bone.

The Achilles tendon is named after Achilles, a warrior in Greek mythology. According to this legend, Achilles's mother tried to make him immortal by dipping him into the sacred River Styx. Unfortunately she held him by the heel, which never touched the water, so the heel did not receive any special powers. It remained vulnerable. Similarly, the Achilles tendon does not have any protection like the patella gives the tendon in front of the thigh. As a result, this tendon is at risk from damage caused by strenuous exertion or from shoes that do not fit properly.

BLOOD FLOW AND NERVES

Surrounding the Achilles tendon and other internal parts of the legs are blood vessels, or tubes that move blood through the body. There are two types of blood vessels: arteries and veins. Arteries carry blood away from the heart, and veins carry blood to the heart. Blood travels along arteries like a car on a highway, making stops to deliver oxygen, nutrients, and other essential things that help to sustain and fuel the legs. That is one reason why the heart rate of a person who is running increases. The leg muscles need more oxygen and fuel, so the heart pumps harder

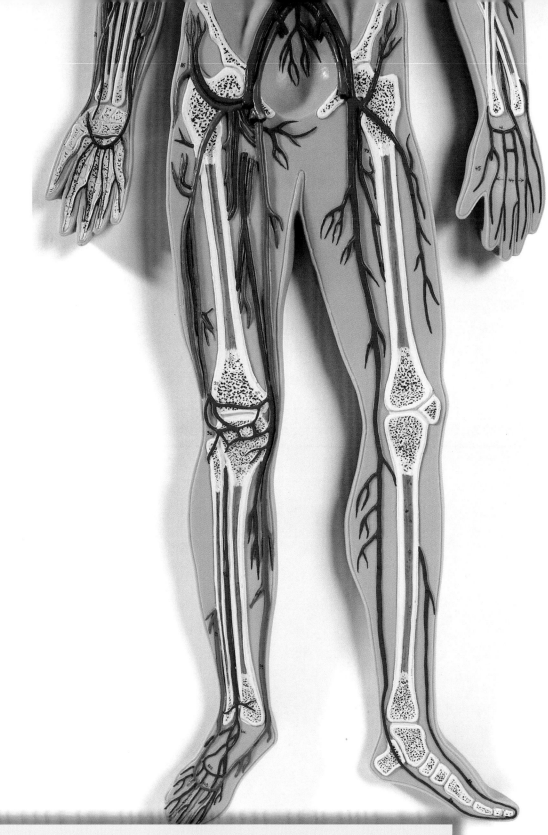

This diagram illustrates blood flow through the lower limbs. The red arteries carry oxygenated blood from the heart to the rest of the body. The blue veins carry deoxygenated blood back to the heart.

to increase the blood supply. Veins then pick up low-oxygen blood that needs reenergizing and deliver it back to the heart, which will pump the blood into the lungs for an oxygen fill-up.

There are many arteries and veins in the legs, each with their own name. The iliac arteries and veins, for example, take care of blood deliveries and pickups from the pelvic region to the thighs. Originating near the knees, femoral arteries and veins control blood that is transported through the lower legs.

Nerves originating from the spine also branch out within the legs. Major leg nerves include the sciatic nerves, which run through the hip bone and into the thighs; the femoral nerves, which—like the femoral arteries and veins—run down the femurs and into the lower legs; and the sural nerves, which carry messages to the feet.

CHAPTER FOUR

THE ANKLE AND FOOT

etween the ankle and the foot is a synovial joint called the ankle. The ankle connects the lower leg to the foot by tendons. The ankle joint allows the foot to move and transfers the body's weight from the foot to the leg, which facilitates both walking and balance. It both absorbs the impact of activity and helps propel the foot and body.

The foot itself lies below the ankle. The front part of the foot, or forefoot, has five digits, which are the toes. The middle part of the foot (midfoot) includes the foot's arch, while the foot's rear portion (hindfoot) includes the heel. Throughout the ankle and foot, there are twenty-six bones, thirty-three joints, and more than one hundred muscles, tendons, and ligaments. A foot is often less than half as big as a person's arm and is not nearly as thick and muscular as the thigh, yet the feet carry the weight of the entire body.

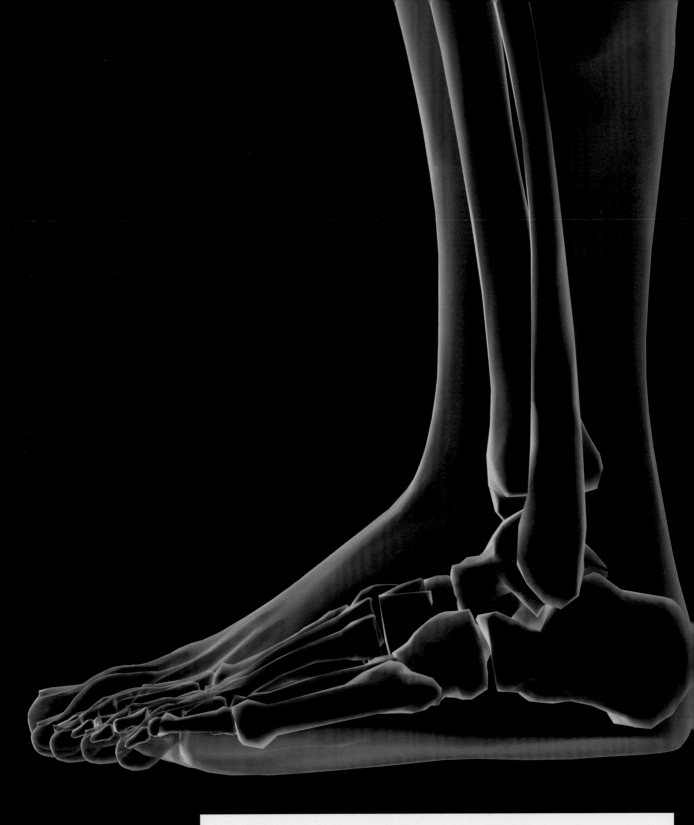

The human foot has twenty-six bones, which form two arches that support the body: the longitudinal arch, along the length of the foot, and the transverse, or mediotarsal, arch, which runs across the foot below the toes.

THE ANKLE

Bones in the feet are relatively soft, compared to those of the thigh and lower leg. This provides greater flexibility and aids in walking. At the top of the foot, the tibia and fibula bones of

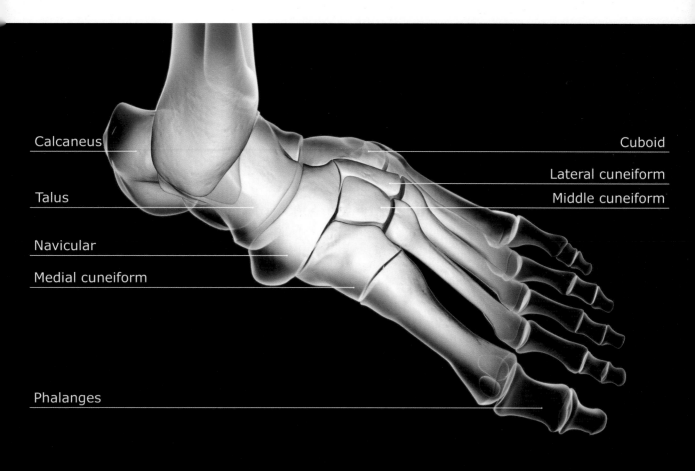

Calcaneus

Cuboid

Lateral cuneiform

Talus

Middle cuneiform

Navicular

Medial cuneiform

Phalanges

This diagram illustrates some of the major bones of the foot, including the talus, which transfers the body's weight from the ankle to the leg.

the lower leg fit into the talus. The tibia and fibula bulge out on either side, forming the medial malleolus and the lateral malleolus. These create the ankle, and they can be easily felt with the fingers.

THE ROLE OF TENDON SHEATHS

The area where the lower leg meets the foot is full of muscle endings and tendons. The reason for so many tendons is that, while the foot contains muscles, most of the muscles that control foot movement are in the legs. This allows the feet to move freely without being weighed down by huge muscles. Imagine, for example, if the thigh muscles were in the foot. People would clomp around with awkward, heavy steps. Because there are so many tendons in the foot, the tendons are enclosed in sheaths.

Tendon sheaths in the foot look a bit like shoehorns. They are located where the foot curves to form the shin. The job of tendon sheaths is to protect the many tendons of the foot from sustaining damage from friction and abrasion. The sheaths consist of a double layer of tissue. The space between the layers, where the tendons lie, is filled with lubricating fluid. The fluid allows the tendons within the sheath to slide back and forth with ease. Given all of the abuse feet take, the tendon sheaths come in handy. For example, think of playing soccer or football. With every kick, the tendons must withstand the forceful blow.

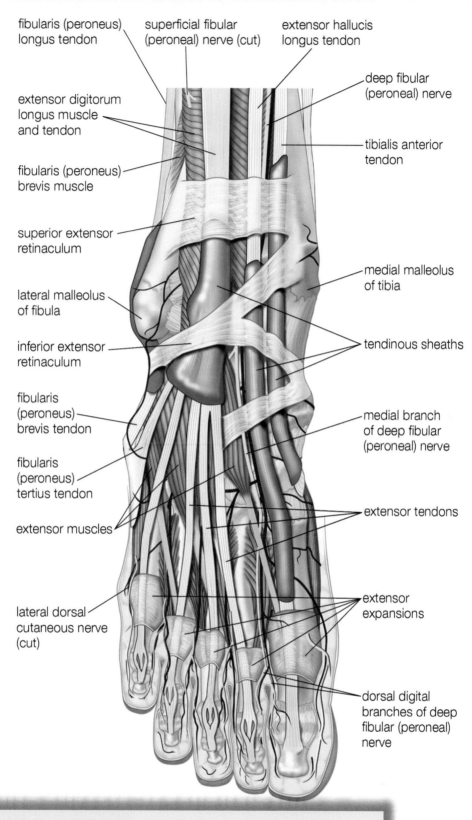

fibularis (peroneus) longus tendon

superficial fibular (peroneal) nerve (cut)

extensor hallucis longus tendon

deep fibular (peroneal) nerve

extensor digitorum longus muscle and tendon

fibularis (peroneus) brevis muscle

tibialis anterior tendon

superior extensor retinaculum

medial malleolus of tibia

lateral malleolus of fibula

inferior extensor retinaculum

tendinous sheaths

fibularis (peroneus) brevis tendon

medial branch of deep fibular (peroneal) nerve

fibularis (peroneus) tertius tendon

extensor muscles

extensor tendons

lateral dorsal cutaneous nerve (cut)

extensor expansions

dorsal digital branches of deep fibular (peroneal) nerve

This illustration shows many of the muscles, tendons, and nerves of the foot. Also marked are tendon sheaths in the foot and in front of the ankle joint. These protect tendons from friction.

Just as athletes sometimes wrap parts of the body with tape, the feet are bound together by broad ligaments. These look like masking tape wound around where the lower leg meets the ankle. These ligaments help to hold the foot's many tendons in place. The fleshy parts under the tendons in the foot consist of skeletal muscles. These give the foot its shape. The skeletal muscles also pull on the tendons at the tip of the foot, which moves the toes.

FIVE DIGITS

The toes on each foot are designed to aid in walking. During a zoo visit, check out what similar digits look like on the feet and legs of chimpanzees and birds. The chimp equivalent of toes actually look more like fingers, which is one reason why chimps like to climb more than humans. Bird legs often have thin sticklike ends, which provide support but are not as good for walking.

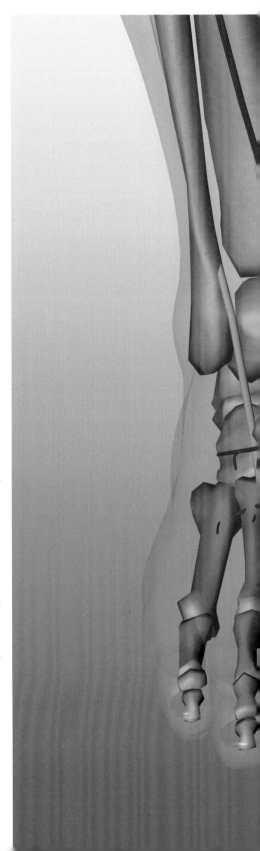

Each toe has joints that help it bend and facilitate smoother walking and motion.

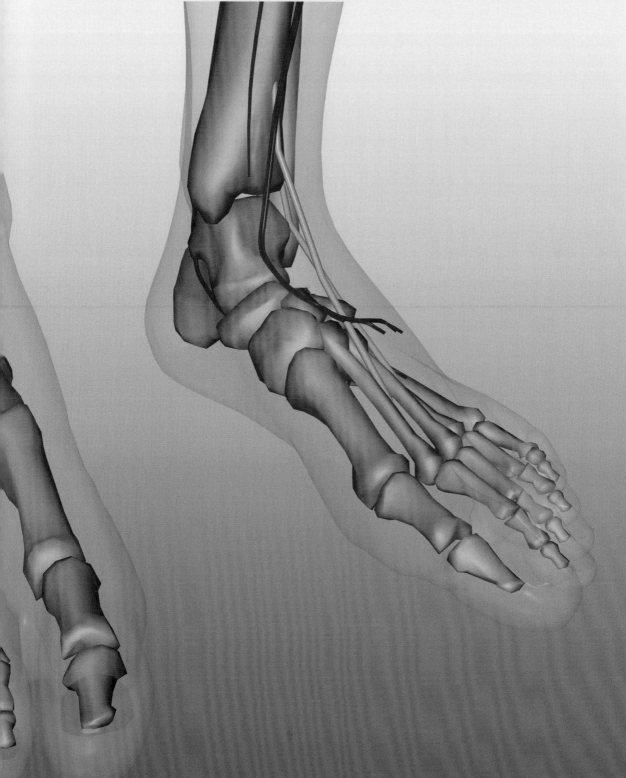

WALKING ON PINS AND NEEDLES

When a foot is held in an awkward position for a long time it can "fall asleep." This often occurs when a person sits on a foot for too long. A foot that is asleep may feel numb. That is because too much pressure blocks sensory nerves. The nerves can no longer send messages to the spine and into the brain, so the foot loses feeling. When the individual stands up and shakes the affected foot around, the nerves gradually recover. During this time, the person will likely feel a tingling sensation—often described as "pins and needles"—as the nerves regain the ability to send and receive messages.

Humans have five toes. The scientific name for the big toe is the hallux. Next to it is the second toe, followed by the third, fourth, and fifth, or little, toe. The big toe has its own muscles, which is why it can move around in several directions. Try moving a big toe now. Now try to move each of the three middle toes by themselves. What happens? The reason it is not possible for the three middle toes to move individually is because they share the same muscles. The little toe, like the big toe, has its own muscles. However, it has a more limited range of movement.

Covering the toes on the outside of the skin are toenails. In the early years of human evolution, people walked barefoot and the toenails wore down by themselves. Now they

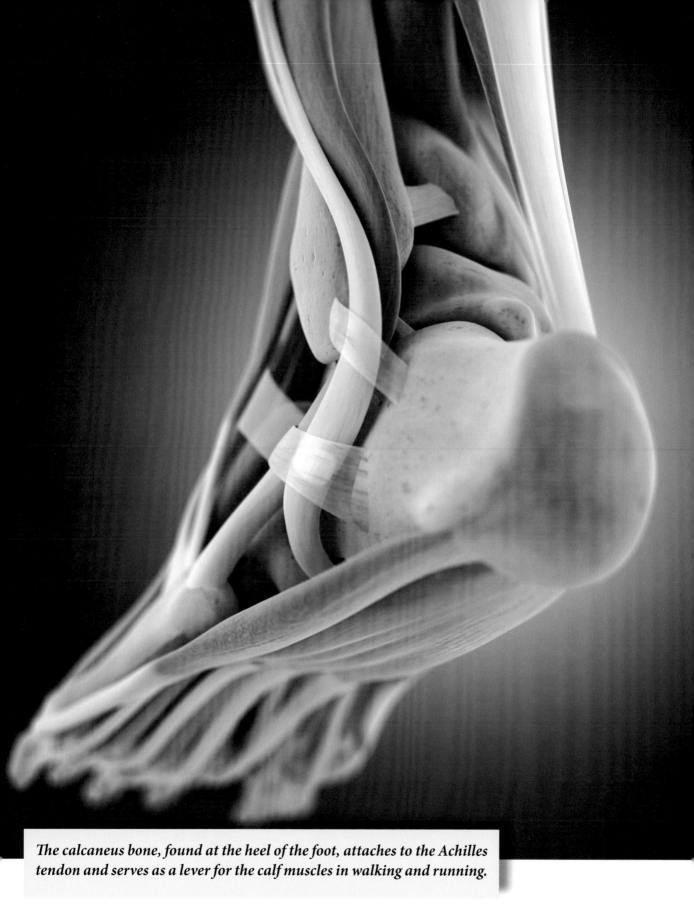

The calcaneus bone, found at the heel of the foot, attaches to the Achilles tendon and serves as a lever for the calf muscles in walking and running.

require regular trimming. The reason this does not hurt is because the nails themselves are dead. Nails are attached to the toes by a root, which does contain living cells.

Below the talus is a large bone called the calcaneus. It forms the heel of the foot. Tarsal bones are the relatively short bones in front of the talus and calcaneus. The metatarsals are longer and are arranged in front of the tarsals. Finally, the toes get their structure from phalange bones.

MOBILITY AND BALANCE

The feet perform many functions, including walking, running, and maintaining balance. Balancing the body on two legs requires a bit of work. This skill comes naturally, for the most part, yet the legs are constantly sending messages to the brain as to what is the best way to stay balanced. Sensory nerves in the feet, for example, let the brain know what kind of surface the feet have to adapt to, whether it is a smooth pavement or a sandy beach. These senses can be fooled, though. With permission, try standing barefoot on a pillow with both arms stretched outward for balance. Now, with a friend nearby to help, place a blindfold over the eyes, lift one leg, and place the arms to the sides. The friend may have to provide balance, as the foot touching the pillow will struggle to keep the body standing upright.

Walking is yet another function performed by the feet and legs that requires skill. Babies cannot walk when they are born.

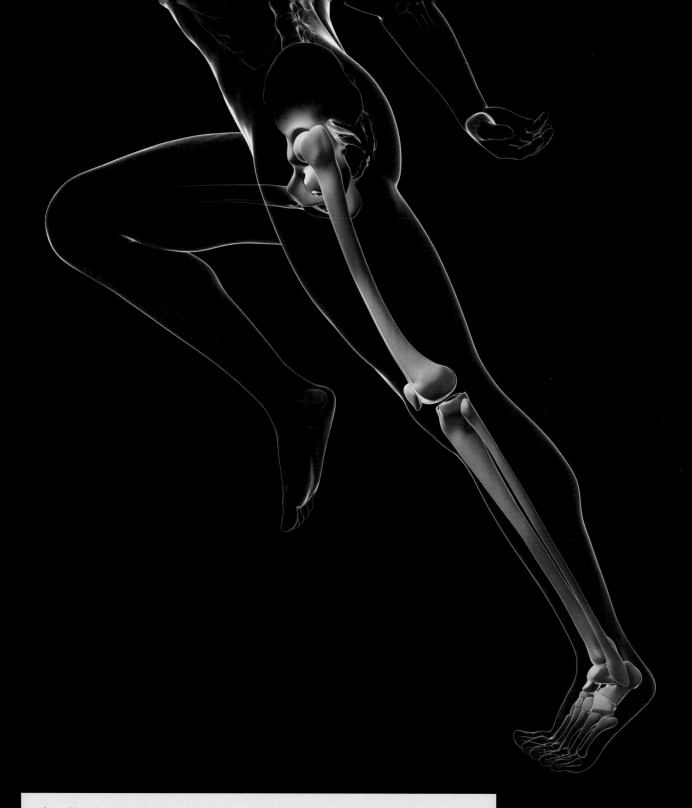

This illustration depicts the major lower limb joints involved in running. Internal support from muscles, tendons, bones, and ligaments, and external support from shoes can help moderate the strain running exerts on the feet and legs.

They have to learn how to coordinate the parts of the body. Coordination is like programming a computer. The brain has to fine-tune the muscles and nerves so that they will work together in unison. When a baby takes his or her first steps, it truly is a special moment because at that point, he or she has coordinated the movements necessary for walking.

Running requires a more advanced form of coordination and a great deal of footwork. As each foot pounds to the ground, the weight of the entire body descends down from the tibia and into the talus. That is one reason why good running shoes provide ample talus, or ankle, support. The weight then pushes forward to the tarsals and metatarsals before it moves backward to the calcaneus. With such a pounding, it becomes evident why so many muscles, tendons, bones, and ligaments are needed in the feet.

Though they are learned skills, walking and running are fairly basic functions. Using the same learning process, people can perform other incredible feats with their feet. Think of track and field athletes who perform long jumps and leap over hurdles. Gymnasts can learn to walk gracefully on a thin bar. Basketball players can dunk the ball with a split-second twist and jump. Ballet dancers can even balance their entire body on their toes. With practice, the limits of foot and leg coordination are virtually endless.

GLOSSARY

ACHILLES TENDON The long tendon that runs from the calf to the heel of the foot.

ACTIN A protein that, along with another protein, myosin, is responsible for muscle contraction.

BALL-AND-SOCKET JOINT A joint, such as that formed by the acetabulum in the hips meeting the femur bone of the thigh, that allows for full rotational movement.

BONE Multilayered hard tissue made primarily of collagen fibers and minerals that provides support and structure to the body.

CALF The back part of the lower leg.

CARTILAGE Protective tissue found in the nose, in the ears, and around the ends of bones at joints.

COLLAGEN Tough protein found in skin, cartilage, and bone.

CONTRACT To shorten and tighten a muscle, which causes the muscle to pull up bones attached by tendons.

FEMUR The longest and heaviest bone of the body that begins at the hip and forms the upper part of the knee joint.

FIBULA A bone located in the lower leg that begins at the lower part of the knee joint and ends at the foot.

HINGE JOINT A joint that allows for back and forth movement, such as the hinge joint at the knee.

JOINT A place where two or more bones meet.

LIGAMENT Firm, bandlike tissue that holds bones together at joints.

MARROW Soft material in the center of bones.

MENISCUS Crescent-shaped fibrous cartilage found between the surfaces of joints, such as that of the knee.

MUSCLE Strong tissue that gives bones and the rest of the body movement.

NERVE A cylindrical fiber that originates at the spinal cord and carries messages to and from the brain.

NEURON A nerve cell, or building block, that makes up nerves.

NEUROTRANSMITTER A chemical substance released by neurons that transmits signals, or impulses, between nerve cells.

PATELLA A disk of bone, commonly referred to as the knee-cap, that protects the tendon at the front of the knee joint.

PHALANGE Of or relating to the bones found in the digits, i.e., the fingers and toes.

REFLEX An involuntary movement performed by the body, usually to protect itself, as exemplified by the knee jerk reflex.

SHIN The front part of the lower leg.

SYNOVIAL FLUID An oil-like liquid that lubricates certain joints, such as those found at the hip and at the knee.

TALUS Commonly called the anklebone, the talus is located just above the heel in the foot.

TARSAL Of or relating to bones found in the foot and ankle.

TENDON A fibrous band of tissue that connects muscle to bones.

TENDON SHEATH Double-layered tissue that protects tendons, such as those located in the feet.

TIBIA The second largest bone of the body, which begins at the lower part of the knee joint and ends at the foot.

FOR MORE INFORMATION

American Association of Anatomists (AAA)

9650 Rockville Pike

Bethesda, MD 20814

(301) 634-7910

Website: http://www.anatomy.org

Members of the AAA include researchers and educators in the field of biomedicine. The AAA is dedicated to advancing the study of biological structures and offers various grants, publications, and other resources to that end.

Canadian Society for Exercise Physiology (CSEP)

18 Louisa Street, Suite 370

Ottawa, ON K1R 6Y6

Canada

(613) 234-3755

Website: http://www.csep.ca/english/view.asp?x=1

CSEP performs research in the areas of health and fitness and sets standards for physical activity and personal training in Canada. Physical activity guidelines, information on trainer certification, publications, and more are offered on the organization's website.

Human Anatomy & Physiology Society (HAPS)

251 SL White Boulevard

P.O. Box 2945

LaGrange, GA 30241

(800) 448-4277

Website: http://www.hapsweb.org

HAPS is dedicated to promoting anatomy and physiology education in high school, colleges, and beyond. The organization sponsors an annual conference and various workshops and offers other resources to members.

Museum of Health Care at Kingston

Ann Baillie Building National Historic Site

32 George Street

Kingston, ON K7L 2V7

Canada

(613) 548-2419

Website: http://www.museumofhealthcare.ca

The Museum of Health Care offers visitors the chance to learn about how disease and other medical issues experienced by Canadians past and present affect physiology. In addition to onsite exhibits, the museum offers online exhibits, including an overview of joints and joint replacement.

Mütter Museum

19 S. 22nd Street

Philadelphia, PA 19103

(215) 560-8564

Website: http://muttermuseum.org

The vast collections of medical specimens, instruments, and models at the Mütter Museum include North America's tallest skeleton and Einstein's brain. The museum also offers many classes to middle school and high school students to allow them to explore anatomy, disease, and more.

National Museum of Health and Medicine (NMHM)

2500 Linden Lane

Silver Spring, MD 20910

(301) 319-3300

Website: http://www.medicalmuseum.mil

Visitors to the NMHM can view various historical medical artifacts and specimens used in American and military medicine. The NMHM also offers workshops that allow visitors to learn more about the human body's anatomy.

WEBSITES

Because of the changing nature of Internet links, Rosen Publishing has developed an online list of websites related to the subject of this book. This site is updated regularly. Please use this link to access this list:

http://www.rosenlinks.com/HB3D/Lower

Ballard, Carol. *Bones*. Mankato, MN: Heinemann-Raintree, 2009.

Calais-Germain, Blandine. *Anatomy of Movement*. Seattle, WA: Eastland Press, 2007.

Colligan, L.H. *Muscles*. Tarrytown, NY: Marshall Cavendish Benchmark, 2010.

Devalier, Frédéric. *Devalier's Stretching Anatomy*. Champaign, IL: Human Kinetics, 2011.

Dicharry, Jay. *Anatomy for Runners: Unlocking Your Athletic Potential for Health, Speed, and Injury Prevention*. New York, NY: Skyhorse Publishing, 2012.

Dimon, Theodore, Jr. *Anatomy of the Moving Body: A Basic Course in Bones, Muscles, and Joints*. Berkeley, CA: North Atlantic Books, 2008.

Floyd, R.T., and Clem Thompson. *Manual of Structural Kinesiology*. New York, NY: McGraw-Hill Education, 2014.

Gilroy, Anne M., Brian R. MacPherson, and Lawrence M. Ross, eds. *Atlas of Anatomy*. New York, NY: Thieme Medical Publishers, 2012.

Haas, Jacqui Greene. *Dance Anatomy*. Champaign, IL: Human Kinetics, 2010.

Hamilton, Nancy, Wendi Weimar, and Kathryn Luttgens. *Kinesiology: Scientific Basis of Human Motion*. New York, NY: McGraw-Hill Education, 2011.

Nelson, Arnold G., and Jouko Kokkonen. *Stretching Anatomy.* Champaign, IL: Human Kinetics, 2014.

Norris, Maggie, and Donna Rae Siegfried. *Anatomy and Physiology for Dummies.* Hoboken, NJ: Wiley Publishing, 2011.

Puleo, Joe. *Running Anatomy.* Champaign, IL: Human Kinetics, 2010.

Rogers, Kara, ed. *Bone and Muscle: Structure, Force, and Motion.* New York, NY: Britannica Educational Publishing, 2011.

Snedden, Robert. *Understanding Muscles and Skeleton.* New York, NY: Rosen, 2010.

Stewart, Gregory J. *The Skeletal and Muscular Systems.* New York, NY: Chelsea House, 2009.

Striano, Philip. *Anatomy of Running: A Trainer's Guide to Running.* Buffalo, NY: Firefly Books, 2013.

Wanjie, Anne. *The Basics of the Human Body.* New York, NY: Rosen, 2014.

INDEX

A

acetabula, 8–9
Achilles tendon, 28, 36–38
actin filaments, 15
ankle
    structure of, 43–44
    what it does, 41
anterior cruciate ligament, 25
arteries, what they do, 38
arthritis, 21

B

ball-and-socket joints, 9–11, 13, 25
bones
    development, 30
    how broken bones heal,
      33–34
    mineral storage, 32
    rejuvenation, 32
bursae, 23, 27

C

calcaneus, 50, 52
cartilaginous joints, 9
coccyx, 8
collagen, 21, 33

E

elastin, 21
exercise, and leg muscles, 36

F

feet
    function of, 50
    pins and needles feeling in, 48
    structure of, 41, 50
femoral arteries and veins, 40
femoral nerves, 40
femur, 6, 9, 11, 18, 20, 23, 28, 40
fibroblasts, 34
fibrous joints, 9
fibula, 28, 43
fibular collateral ligament, 25

G

gastrocnemius muscle, 36
gluteus, 6
    maximus, 13
    meteus, 13

H

hallux, 48
hamstrings, 6, 17
hinge joint, 25–27
hip bone, 7, 8, 9

I

iliac arteries and veins, 40
infants, bone development in, 30

K

knee
        cartilage's function, 20, 21–23
        what it does, 18–20
knee-jerk reflex, 23

L

lateral malleolus, 44
ligaments, what they do, 23–24, 27, 46

M

medial malleolus, 44
menisci, 21
metatarsals, 6, 50, 52
muscles
        how they work, 15
        movement in toes, 48
myofibrils, 15
myosin filaments, 15

N

nerves
        types of, 40
        what they do, 11–12
neurons, 12

O

osteoblasts, 34

P

patella, 25
pelvic girdle, 4, 7–9
peroneus longus muscle, 34–36
phalange bones, 50
posterior cruciate ligament, 25

Q

quadriceps, 6, 25

R

rectus femoris, 13
red marrow, 30, 32
Roentgen, William, 31–32
running, coordination of, 52

S

sartorius muscle, 13
sciatic nerves, 40
soleus muscle, 36
spinal cord, 11, 12, 23
sural nerves, 40
synovial fluid, 9, 10, 21, 27
synovial joints, 9

T

talus, 44, 50, 52
tarsals, 50, 52
tendons, what they do, 17
tendon sheaths, 44–46
thigh
      muscles, 13
      strength test, 15
tibia, 6, 18, 20, 21, 23, 28, 43, 52
tibia collateral ligament, 25
tibialis anterior muscle, 36
toenails, 48–50
toes
      muscle movement in, 48
      structure of, 46–50

V

vastus lateralis, 13
veins, what they do, 38–39
vertebrae, 8

W

walking, coordination of, 50–52

X

X-rays, discovery and development
    of, 31–32

Y

yellow marrow, 32

ABOUT THE AUTHORS

Monica Gill is a writer and editor based in Los Angeles. After receiving a degree in biology, she studied dance and Vinyasa yoga extensively as well as their effects on the human body and the lower limbs, in particular. When not in a dance or yoga studio, she can be found tutoring middle school students in science.

Jennifer Viegas has worked as a reporter for Discovery Channel Online News, as a feature columnist for Knight Ridder newspapers, and as a journalist for ABC News and PBS. She has written several educational books for young adults and, in her spare time, enjoys tennis and other leg-moving sports.

PHOTO CREDITS